I0843943

PREGNANCY HEARTBURN RELIEF- GUIDE ON HOW TO MANAGE HEARTBURN AND ACID REFLUX

BY

IRENE R. STONE

Copyright ©

All rights reserved. No part of this publication may be reproduced, distributed, or transmitted in any form or by any means, including photocopying, recording, or other electronic or mechanical methods, without the prior written permission of the publisher, except in the case of brief quotations embodied in critical reviews and certain other noncommercial uses permitted by copyright law.

Copyright © IRENE R. STONE , 2022.

TABLE OF CONTENT

INTRODUCTION

You anticipated the blown ankles, the morning sickness, and the burgeoning guts. But this burning indigestion? Where 'd that come from?
Heartburn, also known as gastroesophageal influx complaint and acid indigestion, is a burning sensation that begins under your breastbone and moves up your esophagus, a tube linking your mouth to your stomach. These acids can indeed make it all the way up your throat.

In addition to experiencing a burning sensation that can last anywhere between a few seconds and several hours, you may also experience
Feel bloated
Burp a lot
Have a sour or bad taste in your mouth
Have a sore throat
Cough constantly
Although the burrito you had for supper probably didn't help (racy foods can exacerbate heartburn), the burning sensation you are experiencing has more to do with hormones than jalapenos.
So if it's not the burrito, what's causing it?

Still, you 're not alone, If you feel like you have a three- alarm fire dancing in your casket. One study set up that over to 45 of expectant mothers experience heartburn. And if you had heartburn before gravidity, you're indeed more likely to have it during.

Heartburn can fire up, so to speak, at any point in gravidity, but it's most common during the alternate and third trimesters. Experts aren't exactly sure what causes the smoldering, but they suspect it's a three-rounded problem.

Hormones
Progesterone, also called the " gravidity hormone " because it nurtures your womb and the baby inside it, is the leading malefactor behind gravidity- related heartburn.
Progesterone acts as a muscle relaxer. In the case of heartburn, the hormone can loosen the tight muscle(called the lower esophageal cock) that closes your stomach off from your esophagus.
When you eat or drink, the muscle generally opens to let contents into the stomach before shutting tightly. But the surging progesterone situations that do during gravidity can make that muscle slack,

allowing stomach acid to backflow up your
esophagus and indeed into your throat.

Growing baby
As your uterus expands with your growing baby, it
competes for space with some of your other organs.
Like a tube of toothpaste being squeezed, your
growing uterus places pressure on your stomach,
making it more likely stomach acids will unmask
out — especially if your stomach is full.
Your stomach will most probably be compressed as
your uterus expands. This may help explain why
heartburn is more common as you progress through
gravidity.

Slowed digestion
Stomach contents persist longer than usual due to
progesterone. The liability of heartburn increases
when digestion slows and the stomach feels fuller
for longer.
Indigestion (dyspepsia) is a feeling of pain or
discomfort in your stomach, while heartburn is a
burning pain in your stomach and casket caused by
stomach acid.

Heartburn is truly common in gravidity because of hormonal changes and your uterus pressing up against your stomach as your baby grows.
Heartburn is constantly touched off by adipose or racy foods, caffeine, chocolate or citrus fruit juice.
You can try to avoid heartburn by eating small reflections more constantly, eating slowly, not lying down or exercising after reflections and sleeping on several pillows.
There are medicines you can use to control indigestion and heartburn, so see your croaker if your symptoms do n't settle down on their own.

CHAPTER 1

WHAT ARE INDIGESTION AND HEARTBURN

More than half of pregnant women witness severe heartburn, especially in the alternate and third trimesters.

Heartburn, also called acid indigestion, is a vexation or burning sensation of the esophagus(the tube that carries food and liquid to your stomach when you swallow). It's caused by stomach contents that are full (come back over).

Indigestion and heartburn are symptoms that are truly common pregnancy.However, you have an 8 in 10 chance you will witness these symptoms at some point in your gravidity, If you 're pregnant.

A sense of pain or discomfort in your stomach is pertained to as indigestion, occasionally known as' ' dyspepsia. This mainly occurs after eating or drinking.

Heartburn, also known as affluence, is a burning pain in your stomach or casket going up towards your throat. The tube connecting your mouth and stomach, known as the oesophagus, is what causes it to be. The acid irritates the stuffing of your oesophagus, sometimes food might come back over from your stomach into your mouth. A bitter taste in your lingo could also come apparent.

Why do I experience heartburn when I 'm pregnant?

Heartburn may be caused by changes in your hormone situations. One of the gravidity hormones, called progesterone, can relax the muscle that generally holds your oesophagus closed where it meets your stomach. By doing this, you can have food and stomach acid influx up your oesophagus. Heartburn becomes more common as your gravidity progresses. This can be when your uterus(womb) pushes up against your stomach as your baby grows. Also, this forces your stomach's contents up into your oesophagus.
You 're more likely to get heartburn during pregnancy if you 've had a baby before or if you get heartburn when you 're not pregnant.

Causes of Heartburn and Indigestion in gravidity

During normal digestion, food travels down the esophagus(the tube between your mouth and stomach), through a muscular cock called the lower esophageal sphincter(LES), and into the stomach. The LES is an element of the hallway between your esophagus and stomach. It opens to allow food through and closes to stop stomach acids from coming back over.
The LES relaxes enough during acid affluence, also known as heartburn, for stomach acid to climb into the esophagus. This can beget pain and burning in the casket area.

Changes in hormone situations during gestation may make it possible for the LES and other esophageal muscles to relax more frequently. The result is that farther acids may sweat back over, particularly when you 're lying down or after you 've eaten a large mess.

In addition, as your fetus grows during the alternate
and third trimesters and your uterus expands to
accommodate that growth, your stomach is under
further pressure. This can also affect food and acid
being pushed back over into your esophagus.
Heartburn is a typical occurrence for most people at
some point, but it doesn't always indicate pregnancy.
Still, if you also witness other symptoms, similar as
a missed period or nausea, these could be signs that
you need to take a gestation test.

CHAPTER 2

5 Foods That Cause Heartburn During pregnancy — And 5 That Don't

Did you know that certain foods can cause heartburn during gestation?
Help the burn with these smart food suggestions.

During pregnancy, there will be days when all you want to do is reach for your favorite comfort foods, but the alternate you take a bite of that French shindig or eat a sprinkle of chocolate delicacies, your casket feels like it's on fire — that's gestation heartburn. Fortunately, you may be able to avoid the flaming monster of heartburn if you are aware of the items that bring on your symptoms.

Foods that cause heartburn during gestation include acidic foods, coffee and soda pop, alcohol, fried and fatty foods, chocolate, citrus, and racy foods.
We will break down why each food causes heartburn and offer suggestions for backups that will not make you feel like you are breathing fire.

Foods That Can Cause Pregnancy Heartburn

While you can not help the hormonal and physical changes that are known to beget acid reflux and heartburn during gestation, you can avoid some of the utmost driving foods to keep the burn at bay. Then there are five foods that can cause heartburn during gestation.

1. Acidic foods and drinks: Acidic foods can irritate the esophagus and add further acid to an formerly sour situation, worsening heartburn symptoms. Generally acidic foods to avoid include:
    - Citrus fruits like oranges, and grapefruit
    - There is acidity in apples, grapes, blueberries, and pineapple.
    - Red peppers, pickles, onions, both cooked and raw, tomatoes, and onions
    - Citrus authorities like orange juice or lemonade

2. Avoid seasonings that have ginger and other high-acidic constituents.

3. Coffee, tea, and soda pop: More largely acidic drinks that can spark heartburn? Coffee, tea, and soda pop. These cherished drinks are known to coil up the heartburn, and that quality is not limited to the caffeinated performances. In fact, when it comes to these drinks' acidic situations, caffeine is not to be condemned.

- Tip

Do you want to give up your morning mug of joe or glass of OJ? Look for lower acid performances and try to enjoy your drink with a mess or snack to avoid introducing the redundant acid to an empty stomach.

4. Alcohol: Alcohol is largely acidic, meaning it'll do you no favors when you are trying to help heartburn. Indeed Non-alcoholic options of your favorite drinks like non-alcoholic(NA) beers are still largely acidic. Apart from the threat of worsening your gestation heartburn, consuming alcohol during gestation is generally considered dangerous due to its dangerous goods on a developing

fetus. Drinking alcohol during gestation can lead to confinement, birth, and fetal alcohol diapason diseases(FASD), which include endless physical, intellectual, and behavioral disabilities in children.

5. Adipose and fried foods: Fried and adipose foods do not have to be acidic to pack a punch with heartburn. Foods heavy in fat, such as full-fat dairy products, take longer to digest, delaying the emptying of the stomach. And as anyone who has ever dealt with burning indigestion after eating French feasts can tell you, the longer food hangs out in the stomach, the further occasion it has to back up into the esophagus to beget discomfort and pain. To help reduce heartburn symptoms, conclude for slender cuts of meat and low- fat dairy products. When possible, sing rather than frying foods. But if you really want that satisfying crunch that only fried foods can offer, consider trying an air range, which does not depend on oil painting to cook food.

6. Chocolate: Still, we've got some bad news. If chocolate is your go- to special treat.

Research has long shown that chocolate is a
major detector for acid reflux because it
contains acidic characteristics similar to
caffeine and cocoa that can drop the pressure
around Consequently, the esophageal
sphincter loosens up just enough to let
stomach acid back up into the esophagus.
Still, try limiting your input to an occasional
mizzle of chocolate sauce or only two places
of a chocolate bar — and avoid eating it on
an empty stomach, If you can not live without
an occasional chocolate fix.

7. Racy foods: While racy foods can transform a
   dish from ordinary to outstanding, they can
   also cause acid reflux when dealing with
   pregnancy heartburn. The secret to what
   makes foods like peppers so racy is capsaicin.
   Capsaicin irritates mucous membranes,
   including the esophagus, which can lead to
   acid influx. But that is not all Capsaicin also
   slows down digestion, which can complicate
   acid influx. Try using fresh sauces and
   non-pepper seasonings to help flavor foods
   without driving heartburn.

Foods That Will Not Cause Heartburn During Pregnancy

Still, you might have to say farewell to some of your favorite foods(at least for now), but that does not mean you can not enjoy a diet with fun flavors and textures, If you want to avoid gestational heartburn. To help lower your chances of heartburn, try switching out driving foods for these easier- to-condensation options.

1. Dairy Low-fat dairy products, such as yogurt, milk, and crapola, are excellent choices to help prevent acid reflux. Dairy is also a good source of calcium and vitamin D, making it a great pick for gestation. Avoid high-fat options since they take longer to digest and can spark heartburn.

2. Herbal teas like chamomile, gusto, slippery elm, marshmallow root, turmeric, and fennel are all soothing options for battling gestation heartburn. But avoid the peppermint because it can make heartburn symptoms worse.

3. Low-acid foods: Low-acid fruits, such as melons and bananas, are incredibly healthful, easy to digest, and won't make heartburn symptoms worse.

4. High fiber foods High- fiber foods like whole grains, root veggies like sweet potatoes and carrots, as well as green veggies like asparagus, broccoli, and green sap, are excellent options that will not spark heartburn.

CHAPTER 3

Exercise To Relief Heartburn During Pregnancy

1. Heartburn & Diaphragm Pain Relief ways

- What You will Need
- - Exercise Ball
- -voluntary- Scarf
- Belly Sifting: For belly sifting, you will want to use your exercise ball and a scarf(a kerchief or distance can work too)! Support your upper body by using the workout ball. Let the belly drop to the ground while the hips stay high. Make sure the scarf is wrapped comfortably, fully covering the belly. Your mate should lift with their legs, rather than using their upper body. Belly sifting takes pressure off the diaphragm helping to palliate pressure on the stomach and lower esophagus.

NOTE: Avoid this fashion if you have an anterior placenta!

2. Ball Side Body & Diaphragm Stretch: Another exercise ball stretch! Again, you'll use the exercise ball to support the upper body and move into positions that target tight spots. Having the ball will allow you to relax your belly fully and move side to side to find diaphragm pressure.

3. Standing or Wall Hip Flexor Stretch: One of our go-to hip flexor stretches has evolved into this standing diaphragm stretch. use this stretch for heartburn relief too! You'll find another variation of this stretch below.

4. Side- Lying Diaphragm Stretch: Lying on your side while stretching the diaphragm for heartburn relief allows you to gain access to a lesser range of stir. You will want room behind you, in order to extend your leg backward. Do your best to include this heartburn stretch in your morning and/or evening routines.

5. Kneeling hipsterism Flexor Stretch with a Reach: By extending along the entire side body, you can stretch the diaphragm and alleviate heartburn. Taking the arm outflow in this stretch allows you to gain mobility and relieve pressure in the diaphragm.

6. Long Body & Diaphragm Stretch: This is a great option if you do not have an exercise ball handy! analogous to the

7. Exercise Ball Side- Body Stretch, you can gain space in the abdominal area to relieve heartburn and diaphragm pain.

8. Diaphragm Self- Lengthening for Heartburn Relief: Tone lengthening or tone- massage around the lower caricature pen and diaphragm is a unresistant way to find heartburn relief! Follow the caricature pen down and out, spending further time in areas that are tender.

PRO TIP

Massage while you stretch! Lying on your left side positions the stomach so graveness can help in relieving heartburn symptoms. When the left side is down, you can blarney under the caricature pen. We like to use Biofreeze or an embrocation while massage to help with towel drag!

Natural Heartburn Relief

Place 1 teaspoon of chia seeds in a shot glass or small mug. Add water, just enough so the seeds are covered. snappily swallow the seeds. You can use this trick 2- 3 times a day(after reflections is a great time). The seeds end up acting as a hedge for the contents of the stomach and relieves heartburn naturally!

CHAPTER 4

Which heartburn drugs are safe during pregnancy ?

A lot of pregnant women get heartburn, occasionally pertaining to acid indigestion or acid reflux. This condition is generally inoffensive, but it can be veritably uncomfortable. Thankfully, the majority of instances can be successfully treated with home remedies, along with straightforward dietary and lifestyle adjustments.

Numerous women get relief by eating small, frequent reflections and avoiding racy or acidic foods. For those who need fresh help, some tradition and untoward heartburn specifics are considered safe to take during gestation.

Then there are some guidelines to help you understand which heartburn drugs are applicable to use during gestation.(As with any drug, get the okay from your healthcare provider before taking these.)

Can you take Tums while pregnant?

Yes, Tums are safe to take during gestation. In fact, your first line of defense should presumably be these chewable antacids made from calcium carbonate(occasionally just called" calcium" on the marker). Fast, movable , and effective, they may be all you need to handle heartburn. They indeed taste good enough and double as a calcium supplement.

Antacids containing magnesium hydroxide or magnesium oxide – like Maalox, Mylanta, and Rolaids – are presumably safe when used sometimes at the recommended lozenge. But they are not your stylish option while pregnant because they also contain aluminum hydroxide. Aluminum can be constipating and, in large boluses, poisonous.

Bear in mind that swallowing any liquid, indeed the liquid you need to wash down a tablet, will beget your stomach to do what it does naturally produce digestive authorities – including acid, the veritable thing you are trying to reduce. So it's stylish to swallow or bite tablets with as little liquid as

possible when you are having trouble with
heartburn.

All of these antacid drugs work by negating the acid
that is formerly in your stomach and causing you
pain. Chewable and liquid antacids act much more
snappily than tablets because they are formerly
dissolved. You can experiment to see which you
prefer and what works most effectively for you.

Still, talk to your croaker or midwife about whether
you can take fresh or different specifics, If you are
regularly taking the recommended lozenge and are
not getting relief from heartburn.

What about taking Alka- Seltzer while pregnant?
Remedies containing aspirin(similar as Alka-
Seltzer) should be avoided during gestation. Aspirin
may be listed on a marker as salicylate or
acetylsalicylic acid.(Note occasionally aspirin is
recommended for pregnant women, so it's not
always unsafe, but in this case it's not a good idea.)

Also steer clear of sodium bicarbonate(incinerating
soda pop), which is vended as an antacid in tablet
form, and sodium citrate. Both contain lots of salt,

which makes you retain water. And if you are far enough along in your gestation to have gone into a fear trying to remove rings from your blown fritters or looked down in horror at a brace of fluffy ankles, you will understand why that is the last thing you want right now.

Other heartburn drug for gestation

Still, you may want to ask your provider about using a commodity further effective and longer lasting, generally called an acid reducer, If untoward drugs are not helping enough with your heartburn. Rather than negating your stomach acid like antacids do, acid reducers actually stop your stomach from producing the utmost of the acid it typically would.

Acid reducers will not help with the acid formerly in your stomach, so they work stylish when taken before a mess. Some acid- reducing specifics, similar as Pepcid Complete, are a combination of an acid reducer(similar as famotidine) and an antacid(similar as calcium carbonate or magnesium hydroxide), so they can give immediate relief from the acid that is formerly distressing you and reduce farther acid product for over to 12 hours.

Daily use of Pepcid throughout pregnancy is safe to relieve heartburn, and if you still experience symptoms, you can combine it with calcium carbonate chewables like Tums. However, numerous croakers will recommend proton pump impediments or PPIs, If this does not help. These include lansoprazole(Prevacid), omeprazole(Prilosec), pantoprazole(Protonix), and esomeprazole(Nexium)

Some of these drugs are available untoward and others bear a tradition. All are presently considered safe to take during gestation, indeed during the first trimester. Before using any particular medication for your heartburn, however, consult your ob-gyn or midwife. They can give you helpful tips, tricks, and safety guidance.

Symptoms Of HeartBurn

Hormonal changes may beget acid reflux during pregnancy .

The primary symptom of acid influx is heartburn, which is a burning sensation in the middle of the casket. It may accompany a feeling of heaviness or wholeness in the casket or stomach.

A person may be more likely to witness heartburn
After eating a mess or drinking
When lying down
When bending over
Heartburn can affect anyone at any time, but it's particularly common during pregnancy.

Other implicit symptoms of acid influx include
- A bitter taste in the mouth
- Sore throat
- Cough
- Bloating
- Spewing
- Nausea
- Vomiting

CHAPTER 5

What Lifestyle Changes Help Manage Heartburn?

Heartburn, also called acid influx, is when the muscles of your lower esophagus do not work right. This causes food and acids from the stomach to flow back-- or influx-- into your esophagus.
Effects like food and certain specifics can aggravate it. To make symptoms easier

1. Do not go to bed with a full stomach: Eat reflections at least 2 to 3 hours before lying down. Food will have more time to digest and exit your stomach as a result. Acid situations will also go down before you put your body in a position where heartburn is more likely.

2. Do not organize: Eat lower portions at mealtimes, or try to eat four to five small reflections, rather than three big bones .

3. Eat sluggishly: Take time to eat. Put your chopstick down between mouthfuls.

4. Avoid heartburn triggers: Avoid consuming
    meals and beverages that may cause
    heartburn symptoms.

For illustration

- Onions
- Peppermint
- Chocolate
- Potables with caffeine
- Citrus fruits or authorities
- Tomatoes
- High- fat and racy foods

A heartburn journal is a good way for you to figure
out which foods cause your symptoms.

5. Shed some pounds. However, it can help you
    feel more, If you're fat.

6. Stop smoking: The lower esophageal
    sphincter is a muscle in your body that can
    get weakened by nicotine in cigarettes. The
    gap between your esophagus and stomach is
    managed by that muscle. When it's closed, it
    keeps acid and other effects in your stomach
    from going back over.

7. Avoid alcohol: However, try exercise, walking, If you want to decompress after a stressful day.

8. Keep a journal or heartburn log: Jot down when your heartburn hits and the specific effects you are doing when it comes.

9. Wearing loose- fitting clothes can also help.

10. If Your Heartburn Is Worse When Lying Down: Raise the head of your bed so that your head and casket are more advanced than your bases. The bedposts at the head of your bed should have 6-inch blocks underneath. Do not use piles of pillows. You will put your head at an angle that can put further pressure on your stomach and make your heartburn worse.

11. Eat before. Prior to going to bed, try not to eat for at least three hours.

12. If Your Heartburn Gets Worse After Exercise: Time your reflections. stay at least 2 hours

after a mess to exercise. However, you may get heartburn, If you work out any sooner.

13. Drink further water. Have plenitude ahead and during exercise.

14. Spot Your particular Alarms: Some foods and habits generally spark heartburn, while others affect only certain people. Croakers call it influx. You presumably call it heartburn. But whatever it's called, no one wants to witness the unwelcome sensations of heartburn-- a burning casket pain that moves up toward the throat, and an acidic or bitter taste coupled with the sensation that what you just ate is entering your mouth or throat again.

Nearly everyone has had heartburn from time to time-- perhaps at Thanksgiving, after overdosing on lemon and pie, and many spectacles of wine, and also lying around all day watching football. But about 20% of the U.S. population gets an influx at least daily. Some, who have severe, patient heartburn, may have a more serious condition called gastroesophageal reflux complaint or GERD-- which can contribute to a wide range of other health problems, including a precancerous condition called Barrett's esophagus.

Knowing your unique triggers is one way to manage heartburn. After all, although some foods and life habits are common heartburn triggers, they do not affect all people the same way. One person with heartburn can happily eat citrus fruit, while another ends up miserable lower than an hour after a big glass of orange juice.

Then are three ways to start relating to your particular heartburn triggers.

1. Know the Common Causes of Heartburn

There are top foods and actions most generally linked to heartburn

- Eating large reflections, eating later in the day, and eating fatty foods. These" top three" triggers affect nearly everyone who has heartburn.

- Chocolate. This one, unfortunately, is also nicely harmonious, hitting most heartburn victims. Caffeinated beverages like coffee.Caffeine and coffee can cause problems for some people while they don't for others.

- Citrus products, like oranges and orange juice. While caffeine actually induces influx, citrus just mimics the feeling because of its acidity. Garlic, onions, other racy foods and Tomatoes. Both can cause heartburn, although they tend to be more of an issue when they are cooked.

- Alcohol. All alcoholic beverages can cause heartburn, however some people may be more sensitive to red wine than others.

2. Track Your Heartburn Triggers by Keeping a Food Journal: One way to track which of these common triggers affects you most is by keeping a food journal. However, write it down," If you suppose a commodity has touched off your influx." Keeping a food journal can help your croaker determine what is causing your symptoms. But be sure that what you are writing down is really influx.

numerous people mistake other symptoms-- stomach problems and problems in the esophagus-- for influx. There's a group of functional diseases of the GI tract, and influx is one member of that family, but there are others. The typical feeling of influx is a warm or burning sensation in the sternum that moves up toward the throat.However, you may not have influx but commodity differently, If that is not what you are passing.``Write down the symptoms, as well as what you ate and what you did prior, when keeping track of your triggers. Also, note the timing of your heartburn symptoms." Other gastrointestinal conditions, like perverse bowel pattern, don't inescapably produce symptoms right after eating, But with the influx, you will generally witness the heartburn symptoms within an hour after you ate the food that touched off it."

3. Avoid Heartburn With' Clean Slate Eating': What if you go out for Italian food and eat a mess with tomato sauce and red wine, only to witness that familiar burning sensation lower than an hour later? How can you tell if it was

the sauce, the wine, or both? You can't, So the most effective way of changing your personal triggers is to start with a clean slate. "exclude all the foods that are known to beget heartburn from your diet, and also add them back one by one, to find out which bones are causing the most problems for you," You can also minimize the goods of a heartburn-converting food, like chocolate, by eating small quantities, only as part of a lower mess, and not eating too late." You might do fine with a big mess at breakfast but find yourself miserable if you eat a lot at regular intervals, And do not exercise roundly or lie down for a couple of hours after eating. rather, go for a walk. That helps your stomach to empty further." And flashback , you do not have to suffer in silence. However, untoward antacids can help take care of the problem, If you have occasional heartburn that does not trouble you too much. But habitual, worrisome heartburn is a sign that you should see your croaker ." People frequently suppose heartburn is just a commodity they've to live with, But people with diabetes do not go without insulin, and people with high blood

pressure do not go without their specifics. For
some people, heartburn is a habitual
condition and it needs to be treated that way."

CHAPTER 6

How to help and Treat Heartburn During Pregnancy

There are several things you may take to treat and relieve heartburn during pregnancy. There are certain things that trigger it.
You may have heard that if you experience heartburn while pregnant, your child will be born with a lot of hair. While this particular old woman's tale may have some variation, the truth is that heartburn and indigestion can affect any pregnant woman (even if their baby is delivered without a single hair on his or her head).

What Causes Heartburn and Indigestion in gestation?
As with numerous gestation affections, those pesky hormones are the lawbreakers. Gestation hormones decelerate down the muscles in your digestive tract, causing your food to take a while to move through the body, and digestion to decelerate down(this can also cause some muscles to feel bloated). The same hormones also relax the stopcock that connects your

esophagus to your stomach, which can beget food and or stomach acid to come back over into your esophagus and beget that prickly burning sensation. Another factor at play is your growing baby. As your little bone gets bigger and takes up further room in your tummy, your uterus will begin to push up against your stomach. This pressure on the stomach is what makes heartburn indeed more common(and frustrating) the later you're in your gestation.

How Can I Help Heartburn During gestation?

While(unfortunately) there's not a sure- fire way to put a stop to heartburn during gestation, there are a many preventative measures you can take to see if they help make your symptoms a bit more tolerable

- Try to eat a many small reflections throughout the day, rather than three large reflections
- Eat sluggishly, and bite your food well. The lower air that's introduced into your stomach as you eat, the better for your heartburn

- Drink fluids between reflections, rather of on with reflections, to help your stomach from getting too full
- Avoid slithery or fried food, acidic food and drink(similar as citrus fruit or juice), and racy food
- Don't lay down right after reflections(and try not to eat or drink within a many hours of bedtime)

How Can I Treat Heartburn During gestation?

Indeed if you try all of the effects over, heartburn and indigestion can still bother some people. You can try a many effects to get relief during a flare- up

- Drink some milk or consume some yogurt.
- Mix a bit of honey into a glass of warm milk or gusto tea
- To lessen nighttime flare-ups, sleep with your head raised.
- Try an untoward antacid but ONLY after consulting with your provider

Heartburn is serious business, and if it interferes with your ability to eat or sleep, your doctor may be able to recommend a medication that can provide you more relief. The good news is, whether your heartburn is mild or violent, it won't stick around. The maturity of mas finds that their heartburn and indigestion goes down shortly after birth.

TAKING DRUGS DURING PREGNANCY – A GUIDE TO WHAT IS SAFE

When you 're pregnant, there's so much to do, and guarding your own and your baby's health comes top of the list! From what you should be eating and drinking, to what you should and should n't do on a diurnal basis – there are lots of rules, guidelines and advice.

But one of the most important effects to take into consideration is the drugs that you're taking – or may have to take- while you're pregnant. There are some medicines and drugs that, while impeccably safe for most people, should be avoided by pregnant women.

The fact is that numerous drugs – both tradition and over the counter- can have an effect on your baby. They all enter your bloodstream after you take them- also go through the placenta to reach your little bone . utmost will be impeccably inoffensive but, as your future baby's body is still developing, some drugs can have a dangerous effect.

Of course, you should check with your pharmacist or croaker before you take any new medicines and drugs while you 're pregnant – or indeed if you 're planning a pregnancy. immaculately you would check with your croaker previous to getting pregnant if any drugs you generally take are safe to continue during gestation. Still, if you come pregnant and haven't formerly had advice, do check with your croaker as soon as possible.

But it's still good to have an idea of the kind of medicines you can take, what you should be careful of- and what you should be fully avoiding. So, then our companion is on safe drugs to take while you 're pregnant.

1. ANTICOAGULANT medicines, SUCH AS WARFARIN: These are medicines that thin

your blood. They're used to treat heart conditions and are also given to people at increased threat from blood clots or stroke. If you take these medicines in the early stages of gestation also it could be dangerous to your baby's facial and internal development. If your medical condition means that you'll still need to continue anticoagulant medicines the type of drug can be changed to one which is safer during gestation.

2. SODIUM VALPROATE: This is a medicine that's used to treat epilepsy. But exploration shows that it can lead to birth blights and experimental abnormalities if you take it while you're pregnant. However, so that an indispensable treatment can be decided on, If you're taking sodium valproate and are planning a gestation you should speak to your croaker before you stop contraception. Still, if you become pregnant while taking sodium valproate you shouldn't stop taking it, as this could cause your seizures to increase. But you must communicate your GP, Specialist or Specialist nanny incontinently to consider indispensable safer drugs for your condition.

3. ANTIDEPRESSANTS: A lot types of internal health drugs can affect your future baby, so it may be that indispensable treatments need to be set up. But, if you come bad due to not taking your drug that could also harm your child. So, if you get pregnant – or are planning a gestation- while takinganti-depressants, a discussion with your croaker is essential. They will look at the possibility of your current specifics affecting your baby, as well as the pitfalls associated with withdrawing from these medicines. This is particularly important with certain drugs, similar to venlafaxine and paroxetine.

4. ANTI-MIGRAINE DRUGS: Medicines that are specified to help migraine attacks – like ergotamine and methysergide – are associated with an increased threat of confinement and birth, so shouldn't be used when you 're pregnant. Also, a family of medicines known as triptans, which are used to treat migraines, are only recommended for use with medical supervision. communicate with your GP to

bandy how you can manage your migraine
headaches during gestation.

5. ACNE AND PSORIASIS MEDICATION:
    Two medicines used to treat acne and
    psoriasis- called isotretinon andco-cyprindiol
    – aren't safe for pregnantwomen.However,
    which means gels and creams that you apply
    to your skin, similar as benzoyl peroxide and
    antibiotic creams, If you're taking these drugs
    also your croaker will advise you switch to
    safe topical treatments. However, you should
    stay away from any topical therapies that
    contain vitamin A.

6. ANTIHISTAMINES: Antihistamines help
    with dis inclinations similar to hay fever and
    prickly heat rash, but not all antihistamines
    are safe to take during gestation. So, you
    should check with your pharmacist or GP
    before you take them.However, your croaker
    will define a commodity you can take safely,
    If there's a problem with your normal drug.

7. OVER THE COUNTER MEDICINES: You
must still be careful when buying drugs in
shops, or over the counter in a druggist. Some
normal, everyday analgesic drugs – similar to
ibuprofen – can have dangerous goods on
your future baby. Paracetamol is safe to take
while you're pregnant, as there's no clear
substantiation to suggest it could harm your
baby. But you should still take it at the
smallest possible cure, for the shortest time
before stopping. With all over the counter
drugs, it's still judicious to check with your
chemist if they're safe to take while pregnant-
or if planning to get pregnant.

CHAPTER 7

HOW TO GET RELIEF OF HEARTBURN DURING PREGNANCY FAST(USING HOME REMEDIES)

Extended or severe heartburn is a commodity you should talk to your croaker about. Still, for mild to moderate occurrences, there are home remedies for heartburn during pregnancy.However, it's good to know how to snappily get relief of your heartburn, If this condition affects you.

Then are some remedies to try

1. Water (belted throughout the day). While heartburn may make you feel like your chest is on fire, you should n't try to extinguish that fire by gulping water. Drinking too much water too snappily can actually worsen your symptoms. rather, stay doused and reduce heartburn by belting small quantities of water throughout the day.

2. Peppermint. Having a glass of peppermint tea or sucking on sugar-free peppermint delicacies can help relieve heartburn.

3. Ginger. Consuming ginger in tablet form, as chews or by slicing it into thin strips and steeping in hot water for 10 twinkles helps some women get relief. still, use ginger in temperance as large quantities and frequent consumption can bring about condensation.

4. Lemon water. Lemon can help balance your stomach acid and relieve heartburn by promoting the product of corrosiveness and digestive authorities. Try squeezing a many wedges into an altitudinous glass of water and belting on it.

5. Apple cider ginger. An 8-ounce glass of water with a spoonful of apple cider ginger will help balance stomach acid levels and lessen heartburn symptoms. You might discover the most effective heartburn therapy during pregnancy by trying some of these methods.

CONCLUSION

You may have a more serious issue that needs to be addressed if your heartburn frequently wakes you up at night, returns as soon as your antacid wears off, or causes other symptoms (such difficulty swallowing, coughing, weight loss, or black stools).

You might have GERD, according to your doctor. This means that you must manage your heartburn in order to prevent problems like esophageal injury.

Some drugs that lower acid levels may be recommended by your doctor.

H2 blocker medications, which work to stop the creation of acid, seem to be safe.

Proton pump inhibitors are another class of drug used to treat persons with heartburn who don't respond to other forms of therapy.

Talk to your doctor if you have any concerns about the side effects of your medications. Doctors can assist you in managing your symptoms while protecting the health of your unborn child.

www.ingramcontent.com/pod-product-compliance
Lightning Source LLC
Chambersburg PA
CBHW070959260726

48661CB00007B/2755